EASY EXERCISES
FOR
THE OLDER PERSON

GW00683522

MONICA P. FILE, MCSP

Illustrations by
William T. File

EMISSARY PUBLISHING
PO Box 33, Bicester, Oxfordshire, OX26 4ZZ, UK

First published in Great Britain 1999 by
Springfield Books, Witney, Oxfordshire.
Reprinted 2000, 2001, 2002, 2003, 2004

Published in 2005 by Emissary Publishing
PO Box 33, Bicester, Oxon., OX26 4ZZ
Reprinted 2006, 2007, 2008, 2009, 2010

British Library Cataloguing-in-Publication Data.
A catalogue record for this book is available from the British Library.

ISBN: 978-1-874490-76-0

Produced by Manuscript ReSearch (Book Producers)
P.O. Box 33, Bicester, Oxon, OX26 4ZZ, UK.
Tel: 01869 323447
Printed and bound by MWL Print Group Ltd., South Wales

To
My husband,
Bill,
for all the patience and encouragement
he has given me and without whose help
I would not have written this book.

CONTENTS

INTRODUCTION

I have written this book for the individual older person who is living at home, or is perhaps in a nursing or residential home.

I am a physiotherapist of some forty years experience having worked with all types of persons who had many different medical conditions and problems. I have very much enjoyed my work, but particularly my involvement with older people.

I realise how difficult life can sometimes become as one gets older. So, in this book, I suggest a number of simple, gentle, but important exercises to help you maintain your independence and well being. Throughout the book I have presented the material as if I am talking to just one person. I have purposely kept it very straight forward and non-technical, as it is not easy to explain exercises on paper. I also have included a number of "tips" which may help you, as well as the exercises.

When you first read this book, try each movement once or twice. I will explain about the number of times to do each exercise, and how often to do them, in the section headed "General Information" at the end of the book. There is also a complete list of exercises at the end.

Although all the exercises discussed here are not strenuous ones and do not require much more energy than your normal daily activities, if you have any doubt, or are under medical supervision, you must consult your doctor before starting them.

The exercises are a set of very general ones for your whole body. You may feel that some of them may be more beneficial to you than others. If, for example, you have swollen ankles or stiff knees then the leg and foot exercises will help you. If you have difficulty using your arms, then the arm and shoulder exercises are perhaps the ones on which you should concentrate. Perhaps just pick out a few of the exercises which will be of most benefit to you.

There will be some days when you feel a little "under the weather", so don't force yourself to do the more difficult ones. Have a break from them and start again when you feel better.

If you have to have a day or two in bed, you can still do the hand and finger movements. The one where you pull your ankles up and down is also very important if you have to lie in bed.

Just use your common sense. I do hope that the information will be helpful and beneficial to all those who read this book.

WHY DO YOU NEED TO EXERCISE?

Age catches up with all of us, and most of us as we get older, tend to exercise less and less. I don't mean strenuous exercise such as tennis, cycling, or long walks. It is often so much easier to let people do things for us, that perhaps we could do for ourselves. We also don't like to admit it, but we often feel lazy and can't be bothered to do things that require effort. For example, if we drive, it is so much easier to hop into the car, or perhaps be driven to the local shops, rather than to walk.

We also find that some of our joints become stiffer and may be a little arthritic and painful. Our instinct, if our joints are stiff and aching, will normally be to keep still, which will increase the problem.

Our joints have worked very hard all our lives and taken quite a battering with all the daily activities that we undertake. Not to mention the punishment that we have given our bodies with such things as sport, lifting heavy objects, pushing furniture around, gardening, and so on.

All of this means that, because of our lack of regular exercise or movement, over a period of time, our muscles will invariably lose some of their strength. In other words, our arms, back, and legs will become weaker.

You then become trapped in what I call the "vicious circle effect".

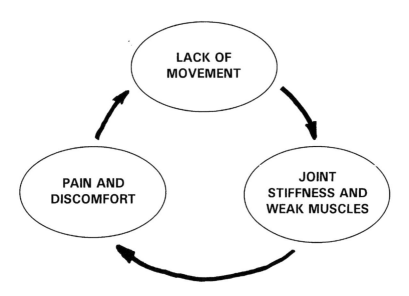

By this I mean that because you are feeling tired, perhaps lazy, or can't be bothered to do something that requires effort, you don't do it. It may be that you have pain on movement and so your instinct will be to keep that part still. To a degree that is necessary, as painful joints need rest, but it is still very important to move your arm or leg as far as you can in each direction. This will help to prevent stiffness. Keeping a joint still means that your muscles have not been used. The muscles become weaker through lack of use and then your joints will become stiffer.

If you are stiff, you will need more effort to perform a certain task, and you can easily say, "No, I think I'll leave it," or else "I'll do that tomorrow!"

In other words we have become trapped in a vicious circle.

One of the results of this "vicious circle effect" is that you might find that you lose your confidence.

You may be frightened of falling, which could increase the vicious circle effect further. When a lot of effort is required it may be tempting not to do much. This leads then to the muscle weakness and stiffness mentioned earlier, which results in a lack of fitness and confidence.

You will be able to help yourself overcome the problems by doing these few exercises regularly. The only way to keep your muscles strong is to exercise them – there is no other way. The exercises will help to keep you fit, build up your confidence, and keep you independent.

The exercises that I have included in this book are all done with the idea of keeping yourself as fit as possible and are not for a specific condition or a particular problem that you may have.

I am sure that if you do have a specific condition, or problem, that your doctor will be helping you. Maybe the doctor or another member of the medical profession – perhaps a nurse or a physiotherapist, is already advising you.

I have explained the exercises in detail and have included a list of them at the end of the book.

These exercises are all performed when you are sitting down. They are all very simple but I have chosen them because they are easy and also very beneficial.

STARTING THE EXERCISES

As you are sitting down, you are very safe and will not have to worry about falling. Start with sitting well back in your chair, and sitting as straight as you can.

BREATHING

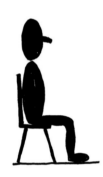 I suggest that you start with deep breathing. This is very important. As the pace of your life has become slower, you do not often have the need to breathe deeply. Your lungs, therefore, are unlikely to be being used to their full capacity, and you will tend to take shallow breaths. This means that you are not getting the boost that extra oxygen will give you, which is vital to make all your systems work as well as possible.

There are many small joints in the chest, for example, where the ribs are attached to the breastbone (or sternum, to give it the medical name). The ribs are also attached to the bones of the spine (the vertebrae). So you can see that it is very important to keep these tiny joints in good condition, as well as all the larger, more obvious joints. Even these tiny joints can become stiff, and the movement effected by the deep breathing will help to prevent this.

Now, sitting straight, take as deep a breath as you can, filling your chest with as much air as possible. Try to make the air fill the lower part of your chest. When you are doing these deep breaths, breathe slowly in through your nose, and breathe out through your mouth.

It is important to take no more than three deep breaths at a time. You will probably find that if you take more, you will feel dizzy. The reason for this is rather technical, but put simply, it is because the carbon dioxide level in the blood is altered. So, no more than three deep breaths at a time. Take a few normal breaths and then another three deep ones.

NECK MOVEMENTS

Most of us lose some of the movement in our necks as we get older. When you think of it, our heads are very heavy and are balanced on our necks. The neck is made up of very small joints. These joints take a lot of wear and tear because we work them very hard. It is therefore very common for our necks to become a little stiff and to lose some of their movement. Heads also have a tendency to drop forward when dozing in an arm chair, which increases the strain on your neck.

Again, see that you are sitting as straight and as tall as you can in your chair. We will do two gentle neck movements.

1. Firstly, just straighten your head so that it is quite level. Then see if you can "tuck your chin in". Relax and try again, keeping your head level. It's as if you are making a double chin.

2. Next, try turning your head to look over your right shoulder, taking it as far as you can. Then gently turn it to the other side. Do this two or three times providing it does not make you dizzy. If it does – stop.

ARM EXERCISES

As you are probably doing more sitting these days and not using your arms as much as in the days when you were perhaps looking after a family, decorating, driving, gardening, or playing sport, your shoulders are not being used as much.

SHOULDER EXERCISES
1. Start by lifting or shrugging your shoulders up towards your ears, and then lowering your shoulders. Don't drop them quickly; just bring them down gently. If you drop your shoulders with a jerk, you will put strain on your neck and all the muscles around your shoulders.

2. Now, just brace your shoulders, pulling them back to give yourself a good stretch across the upper part of your back.

Most of what you do tends to be bending forward or looking down, and you rarely have to stretch back. This is a very good exercise to do for your head and shoulders and it also helps to expand your chest, which is very beneficial for reasons that I mentioned previously.

We will do some hand movements next.

HAND EXERCISES

1. Bend your fingers as tightly as you can. Make a fist and then stretch your fingers out again making your hand as flat as possible. It is very easy to do and again this simple exercise is so important. Your fingers and hands are made up 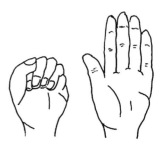 of so many tiny joints and can quickly become stiff if they are not exercised regularly.

Many of you will not be doing as much as you used to so your hands are not being used the same amount. It is essential to keep the strength of your hands for ordinary tasks, such as doing up and undoing buttons, writing letters, cleaning teeth, turning taps, opening doors and so on.

Hands, when relaxed, tend to curl up; so it is particularly important to flatten them and give them a good stretch. It is also very surprising how even our hands lose their muscle strength when not used a lot. I always think of my father who was a dentist and therefore had very strong hands (he needed the strength to do the extractions!). When he became old and less able, even his hands became thin and lost their "padding". This was because the muscles in his hands were not being used.

Back to the exercises!

2. Now bring your thumb across to touch the tip of your little finger, and then stretch it back to make your hand flat. Next touch your fourth finger with your thumb and bring it back. Now touch your middle finger and back. Now bring your thumb to touch 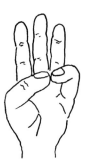 the tip of your index finger, then flatten your hand.

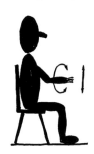 3. Next your wrists – move your whole hand up and down, bending from the wrist. Next make a circle with your hand, just going round and round. Then circle in the other direction.

4. This time, straighten your fingers and then try to spread them out (in other words separate them). Relax, and spread your fingers again.

5. Another good way to keep your lower arms supple is to bend your elbows and tuck them into your sides and turn your hands over and up, over and up.

ELBOW AND UPPER ARM EXERCISES

You may prefer to do these exercises with either one arm at a time or with both arms together. Do which ever is easiest for you, as it doesn't really matter. Perhaps just pick out one or two exercises.

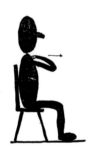

1. Touch your shoulder with your hand, now stretch your arm in front of you until it is straight. Again, touch your shoulder and now straighten your arm. When you are sitting, lying, or relaxing, your arms are almost always bent so it is very good to give them a regular stretch.

2. Bring your hand behind your neck and if you can, creep your fingers down your back a little way. Now stretch your arm forward as though you were reaching for something from a shelf.

3. Next, touch the top of your head and pretend that you are combing your hair.

4. Can you lift your arm out to the side so that your arm is level with your shoulder?

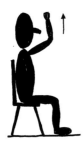 5. Another exercise for your arm is to reach up to the ceiling, taking your arm up as high as it will go, and bring your arm down. Do this with your elbow bent, as if you were pushing up a box onto a high shelf.

You may find this movement easier to do with one arm, and to help it with the other one, especially when bringing it down. I will explain.

If you are lifting your left arm, put your right hand just above and at the back of your left elbow to help lift your left arm. This will take some of the weight off your arm and makes it a little easier. Keep your hand in that position as you bring your arm down.

Repeat with the other arm.

6. A shoulder exercise, that combines all the movements, is to put your hands on your shoulders, and now make a circle with your elbows. You should do this upwards and backwards. This is known as "elbow circling". If you can, do both arms at the same time. As you bring your elbows up and back, give a good stretch across the upper part of your back. It may hurt at first, but does a lot of good to your back.

TRUNK EXERCISES

Just one or two gentle exercises for your back and tummy, that is, the trunk.

1. Again sit as straight as you can – with your feet on the floor. Just gently lean forwards, as far as you feel that you are able, at the same time keeping your back as straight as you can. Stay forwards for a few seconds and pull yourself up so that you are straight again. Do this slowly and very carefully.

2. Next, put your hands by your side and, if you are sitting in an armchair, try and put your arms over the side of the chair, then gently lean to one side going as far as you are able. Straighten up and then lean over to the other side.

LEG EXERCISES

This is a very important section because these simple exercises will keep your legs and feet as strong as possible. This is vital for walking, getting up out of a chair, getting on and off the loo, in and out of the car, etc.

Starting with your feet. It is quite surprising how stiff and awkward feet can feel. Our feet are made up of 26 bones so there are many joints and a number of muscles, which can also become weak.

When you are walking, always try to walk by putting your heel down first. That is a normal walk. It's very easy to get into the habit of shuffling your feet and not using them correctly. They will then stiffen and that will make walking more difficult for you. So, remember when walking, *heels down first.*

FOOT EXERCISES

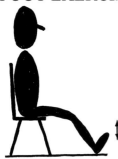

1. Stretch your legs out in front of you, with your feet resting on your heels. Now, keeping your heels on the floor, pull your feet up towards you as far as you can – you might feel a stretch in your calf muscles.

Now push your feet down to the ground. It is just a simple up and down movement bending and stretching your ankles.

This is a very good movement as it helps the circulation in your legs. If you are having to do a lot of sitting about, the circulation (the movement of your blood) can become rather slow. This simple exercise is going to help the flow of blood and will have many beneficial effects.

2. Now, doing one foot at a time, make a circle with your foot, as big a circle as you can. You can either do this exercise with your heel resting on the floor, or better still lift your leg off the floor before circling your foot round. Good, now do it the other way round. This exercise is also very good as it keeps your ankle mobile and also uses the muscles of your legs and feet and again will improve the circulation.

3. Another simple exercise for the feet is bending and stretching just your toes.

KNEE AND HIP EXERCISES

The main muscles that work on our knees are all large and bulky. Surprisingly enough they quickly waste and lose both their bulk and strength. Muscles waste (or become weak) if they are not used, or if there has been an injury to the joint on which they work. Think of the sportsmen who so often injure their knee joints whilst playing. They find that their big thigh muscles will lose their bulk within a matter of hours. This can happen to a lesser extent if you twist your knee or perhaps trip and hurt it.

Once that has happened, the knee joint has lost a lot of its protection and support. The joint is then more likely to become damaged and will probably cause pain and discomfort. This will make you walk badly and cause extra strain on your back.

The big group of muscles in the front of the thigh is called the quadriceps – commonly called the quads, as there are four muscles in the group which all work together. We will concentrate mostly on these muscles, but there are others that are also important.

1. To strengthen your knee muscles – and especially your quads - sit straight in your chair with your feet on the floor. Lift one leg from your knee until the leg

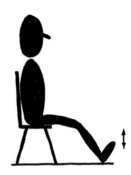

is as straight as possible. Hold it for a few seconds, then lower it slowly. Do the same movement with the other leg. Keep doing this simple movement with alternate legs. You may find it pulling your knees a little but with practice that feeling should get easier. Don't give up just because it hurts a little, or is difficult!

2. Now, a slightly more difficult one for you, which uses some of your hip muscles. Lift your lower leg until your knee is straight (as in number I, above). Then move your whole leg a little to the side and back. Put your leg gently down. This is a stronger movement, so try this one when you are used to doing the simpler up and down movement.

3. Now try marking time with your legs – still in the sitting position – up and down, up and down.

GENERAL INFORMATION

I have suggested a number of simple exercises for you to do in your own home, and I will explain how often you should try and do them.

Start by doing each exercise 3 times. Do this once a day.

By doing this, your muscles and joints will become accustomed to the movements. You will find that all these movements become much easier with regular practise, and that you will also be able to increase them gradually.

By the end of the first week, do each movement 5 times, if you feel able to.

After about 2 weeks, when your joints and muscles are used to the movement, perhaps try to increase the number, slowly working up to 8 times over a period of a month. If you do manage 8 times, have a short rest after 4 and then do another 4.

Don't forget that the head and neck movements and also the deep breathing should only be done 3 times each.

For the first few times, you might experience a little soreness or stiffness in your muscles and joints. This is very normal and is nothing to worry about, and may come on an hour or so after you have stopped, or even the next day.

The walker, or sportsman will experience the same feeling – it's just the body reacting to doing something different, and will lessen as you practise the exercises.

You might like to try these exercises in the morning when you are fresh. Maybe you will find that you like to do some of them twice a day after a while.

You can alter them or vary the order, even miss some out, but if you can, aim to do each movement 8 times, then after a while, you will feel the benefit.

The secret is <u>little</u> and <u>often</u>.

Another important thing to remember is that you don't always have to have a specific exercise session.

If you are watching television or sitting reading, you can move your feet up and down, or lift your legs at the knee two or three times. You can squeeze and stretch your fingers, stretch your arm up towards the ceiling a couple of times. Take two or three deep breaths. Look over your shoulder.

Again the main way to help yourself is to do these exercises <u>little</u> and <u>often</u>.

When doing them, always go to the limit of the range of the movement. I will explain what that means.

As an example, I will use a shoulder movement. Try lifting your left arm up towards the ceiling, doing it with your elbow bent and just pushing gently upwards. Take your arm as far as possible and then, see if you can take it just a tiny bit further. You will find that it will always go just a fraction. In time and after practice, those fractions of an inch will add up and you will find that you can move your arm more easily and a little higher. This applies to all the movements – hands, feet and knees. You will find that you have increased your range of movement – that is, your joints move further and you have increased the strength of your muscles.

HELPFUL TIPS

COMFORT FOR THE NECK AND SHOULDERS

It is often a good idea to have a pillow, or large cushion, on your lap or at your side when you are sitting just relaxing or watching television. You then place your arms on the pillow and your arms and shoulders will be more relaxed. The pillow will take the weight of your arms, which will then relieve strain on your shoulders and also your neck. This is particularly important if you have any pain or discomfort in your arm or neck and is well worth trying. It is a small tip, but can bring a lot of comfort to painful necks and shoulders.

When you are sitting in your easy chair, assuming that it has a high back, try to rest your head against the back of the chair. A very small soft cushion or towel behind your neck will give some support. This will give those neck joints and muscles a chance to relax. It refreshes your neck and makes it easier for the muscles to continue doing the work of supporting your head.

GETTING UP FROM A CHAIR

If you are sitting in a chair, especially a soft or low one, it's not always easy to stand up, and you may have become stiff just because you have been sitting in the same position.

Try to remember before you attempt to stand, to bend and stretch your ankles at least twice. Also, lift up one leg at a time and stretch it out (as we did in the exercises). This prepares your legs for taking your weight.

Now move to the front of the seat. Bring your bottom forward, as it is extremely difficult to get out of a chair if you are sitting well back.

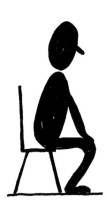

So,

Wriggle forwards

Bring your feet back as far as you can – again, it is very difficult to get up if your feet are well in front of you.

Now lean forward and push up to a standing position. You might need to push on the arms of your chair or perhaps put your hands on your knees.

Once you are up, <u>always</u> get your balance before you move and start to walk. Just stand still for a few moments to make sure that you are steady. This is most important.

So,
1. Move to the front of the chair.
2. Pull your feet back
3. Lean forward.
4. Stand
5. Get your balance
6. Walk

Don't forget, <u>if you feel unsteady,</u> or wobbly when you walk, <u>just stand still</u> for a few seconds <u>until you feel steady and safe.</u>

PREVENTION OF SORENESS OF YOUR LOWER BACK

For someone who is sitting still for most of the day, there is the risk of getting quite sore at your lower back – your "seat area".

To prevent this, try tightening your seat muscles and relaxing. Do this about 4 times whenever you think of it. This is very important and allows the muscles to be "refreshed" by the improvement in the circulation that this simple exercise will cause.

Try to stand up every hour, even if you don't need to go out of the room, taking great care as you do this that you do not overbalance. This will also help prevent the soreness in your seat area, as well as keeping your muscles strong. Follow the guidelines in "Getting up from a Chair" in the previous section.

GETTING UP FROM YOUR BED

When you get out of bed in the morning, or even if you need to get up in the night, sit on the side of the bed for a few seconds before you stand up. This makes a lot of sense, as you have been lying down and then suddenly changed to a sitting position. Many people find that they feel slightly giddy for a short time when they first sit up, so just give yourself time.

While you are sitting on the edge of the bed, and before you stand, just lift up one leg and then the other one, two or three times.

Many people say "Oh, I don't have time to do exercises then" – it is not an exercise session, and it just takes a few seconds. It prepares your legs to take your weight, and just makes you able to stand more safely. Whenever you are walking, if you feel unsafe or giddy, just STAND STILL AND GET YOUR BALANCE – and then start to move carefully.

CONCLUSION

I have tried to suggest very simple exercises for you that I do hope will help a lot. It will be an effort to do them. It is always so easy to think "well, I won't do them now, but I will do them later" – and later never comes! Set aside a time for the exercises. Try making them a part of your daily routine, like brushing your hair or cleaning your teeth.

You really will benefit from doing them and they will help you to stay fit and healthy and help to maintain your independence. I wish you the best of luck, and do enjoy your exercise sessions.

LIST OF EXERCISES

DEEP BREATHING
Take a deep breath, slowly breathing in through your nose, and breathe out slowly through your mouth.
   3 times only (No more at a time).

NECK MOVEMENTS
1. Try and make a double chin.
2. Look over your left shoulder - then bring your head straight.
3. Look over your right shoulder – then bring your head straight.
   3 times only for each movement. (No more at a time)

ARM AND HAND EXERCISES
1. Shrugging shoulders up towards your ears and lowering gently.
2. Brace your shoulders – pull back.
3. Bending and stretching fingers – i.e., making a fist.
4. Bring thumb across to touch tip of little finger, then stretch it back. Repeat this touching each finger in turn.
5. Spread out your fingers.

6. Move whole hand backwards and forwards from your wrist.
7. Making a circle with your hand in both directions from your wrist.
   Up to 8 times for each movement.

SHOULDER AND ELBOW EXERCISES

1. Touch your shoulder with your hand, and then stretch your arm out in front.
2. Put your hand behind your neck – stretch your arm forwards.
3. Touch the top of your head, and then reach up towards the ceiling. Bring your arm down.
4. Lift your arm out to the side and lift it as high as you can.
5. Tuck your elbows into your sides, and turn your lower arms and hands over and up.
6. Elbow circling.
   Up to 8 times for each movement.

TRUNK EXERCISES

1. Lean forwards as far as you can. Come back and sit straight.
2. Lean first to one side and then the other.
   Up to 6 times for each movement.

EXERCISES FOR THE FEET
1. Pull your feet up as far as possible. Then point your feet down. Repeat up and down.
2. Ankle circling – both directions.
3. Bending and stretching your toes.
   Up to 8 times for each movement.

EXERCISES FOR THE KNEES
1. Lift one leg up to straighten leg. Put it down slowly. Repeat with other leg.
2. Lift and straighten your leg. Move the whole leg to the side and back.
3. Marking time – i.e. lifting alternate legs with knees bent (movement from the hip).
   Up to 8 times for each movement.

AND FINALLY,
Change the order of the exercises a little – you probably won't want to do four types of shoulder movements, one after the other. Perhaps just choose 2 or 3 movements one day, then try different ones next time. Change to the leg exercises to give your arms a chance to recover and revive from all the hard work that you are making them do!

There are obviously many more varied and perhaps more difficult exercises that you could do, but I have deliberately kept these simple.

Do take care when you are doing any of these movements and always make certain that you are sitting in a comfortable and well-balanced position. Don't forget that after doing the exercises the first few times that you may feel some reaction. Your joints may feel a little stiff and possibly your muscles a little sore. It will wear off after a few sessions – it does not matter at all and just shows that you have been doing the exercises well.

There may be a time when you are not able to do any exercises. When you come to start again you will quite likely experience some reaction, as you did when you first started. It's only the muscles and joints becoming used to moving again, and is nothing to worry about.

You really will feel the benefit of these simple movements if you make yourself do them regularly.

If you feel able to move more easily, you will also feel generally fitter and more confident. You will feel more positive and cheerful about life. So do try. Remember, I say it again – LITTLE AND OFTEN!

END

LAUGHTER — THE BEST MEDICINE

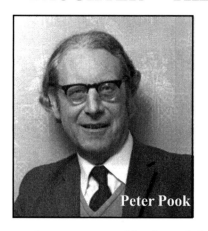

Peter Pook

PETER POOK, brillian wit and author of more than twenty funny books, was, at various times in his life, boxer, foot-baller, bank clerk, diver, Royal Marine, Indian Navy Lieu-tenant, antique dealer, estate agent, car dealer, schoolmaster, lecturer, author—and laugh-master par excellence.

His fans range from nine to ninety and letters are still being received from all over the world.

In response to public demand, Emissary have now published all the Peter Pook novels into paperback, and, in the process, have added a new generation of Pook readers to his growing army of fans. (See Page 42). The following testimonials give an insight into the magic of his work.

A fan from Auckland in New Zealand, wrote:

"You're a bloody beaut. I had to lock myself in the bathroom to read, to keep my wife, son, and mother-in-law from abusing me for disturbing their telly-watching by rolling on the floor and crying with laughter."

A Middlesbro' reader wrote:

"I had a nervous breakdown a while ago. I came home from hospital so very depressed and my husband thought I would never smile again—until I read your books."

Mr. A. of Bristol wrote:

"I am an avid reader of Pook books . . . if only they were available in p.b. I should buy whole sets to send as presents."

And a courageous Mr. Mundy wrote:

"Hi, I thought you would like to know that I was a great Peter Pook fan, and his book .. *Pook in Business* actually changed my life. 28 years ago I gave up my job on the railways to become a self employed .. Antique Dealer.

It changed my life and I owe it all to Peter Pook and his advice in the book and his attitude to life . Regards.... Peter Mundy. p.s...I even started to write down my own adventures in the Antiques business." (May, 2008)

BANKING ON FORM

The problems confronting young Pook as he struggles to combine the art of Banking with sex, body-building and a football career are told in fast tempo and with dry humour.

In the process, to the lay reader's delight and edification at least, Pook reveals the mysteries of the British banking system; becomes entangled in the night life of Paris; develops into the strongman of the financial world; plays soccer on the blood-feud principle, and antagonises every person he comes in contact with—including himself.

But it is all good clean fun, and the laughter which will follow the earnest young man through his hectic career will win him plenty of friends among readers—at any rate outside the ranks of bankers.

POOK IN BOOTS

Leaving the Bank, Pook continues his aggressive career in the Royal Marines, where he mixes with earls and orphans—leading them all cheerfully to perdition, willingly aided by the smallest Marine on record, the Hon. Lesley Pilkington-Goldberg.

Opposing Pook and his dislike of discipline is that magnificent character Sergeant Canyon—fifteen stone of bad-tempered Saxon warrior—whose epic encounter with Pook in the Unarmed Combat Class is still remembered with awe by those who saw it. Also running through the story is the love-interest of Pook's girl-friends, and his encounters with the shrewd tactician Lieutenant Tudor, all of which contribute to making this another roller-coaster of hilarity.

POOK IN BUSINESS

Pook lets us share in the thrills and nightmares of acquiring one's first shop, and opening it to see if the public will actually pay money for the debris of the past. Readers will delight in his advice about how to buy antiques, both from the auction sales and privately, and how he finally solved that unique paradox of the trade—"Any fool can sell it, but it takes a smart operator to buy it."

EMISSARY PUBLISHING, PO BOX 33, BICESTER, OX26 4ZZ

NEW EDITION PETER POOK ORDER FORM—*Cover designs by Richie Perrott*

NAME (Block Capitals)..

ADDRESS (Block Capitals) ....

....

....

POST CODE:...................................Tel. (In case of query) ....

QTY	ALL PETER POOK TITLES £8.50 each (includes p&p.)	TOTAL £
....	Banking on Form	....
....	Pook in Boots	
....	Pook in Business	
....	Pook Sahib	
....	Bwana Pook	
....	Professor Pook	
....	Banker Pook Confesses	
....	Pook at College	
....	Pook's Tender Years	
....	Pook & Partners	
....	Playboy Pook	
....	Pook's Class War	
....	Pook's Tale of Woo	
....	Pook's Eastern Promise	
....	Beau Pook Proposes	
....	Pook's Tours	
....	The Teacher's Hand-Pook	....
....	Gigolo Pook	
....	Pook's Love Nest	
....	Pook's China Doll	
....	Pook's Curiosity Shop	....
....	Marine Pook Esquire	
....	Pook's Viking Virgins	....
TOTAL		**£**

N.B. Add £1.50 per book for overseas surface mail; £3.00 per book for overseas airmail: cheque should be in sterling and drawn on an English Clearing Bank. Emissary reserve the right to change prices without notice: Tel. 01869 323447 for clarification.